Published By Nicholas Thompson

@ Bryan Horton

Wheat Belly Diet: 100+ Best Wheat Belly Diet to

Lose Weight and Lower Blood Pressure

All Right RESERVED

ISBN 978-1-990666-92-6

I0558144

TABLE OF CONTENTS

Coconut And Chocolate Tart

Ingredients:

- ¼ cup of coconut oil you can also use butter; melted

- 14 oz of canned coconut milk you can also use heavy cream

- 8 oz of 100% chocolate

- 3 eggs separate the egg whites

- 2 ½ cups of shredded coconut unsweetened

- ¼ cup of walnut or pecan meal

- 2 teaspoons of ground cinnamon divided

- Sweetener equivalent to a cup of sugar divided

- ½ teaspoon of vanilla extract

Directions:

1. Preheat your oven for 350 degrees F.

2. Grease a 9-inch size pan.

3. In a separate bowl, mix together almond flour, coconut, ½ teaspoon of cinnamon, ¼ cup of sweetener and oil. Mix them well. Transfer to the greased pan and spread them evenly. Bake for about 10 minutes or until the edges of the dough are already browned. Remove from oven and let cool.

4. Meanwhile, heat coconut milk and chocolate on a medium sized pan. Heat on medium flame until the chocolate is completely melted. Stir remaining sweetener. Do not overheat. Once d2, remove from the heat and set aside.

5. Whip the egg whites in a bowl until it forms stiff peaks. Using a mixer, blend yolks, cinnamon and vanilla. Add the chocolate

mixture slowly until it becomes evenly
combined.

6. Pour the chocolate mixture over the crust and
   bake for another 15 minutes. Remove from
   the oven and let cool. Refrigerate and let it
   set.

7. Serve and enjoy!

Bbq Crockpot Pork

Ingredients:

- 2 tbsp. of ground cumin

- 1 tbsp. of white pepper, ground

- 1 tbsp. of black pepper, ground

- 2 tsp. of cayenne pepper

- 1 tbsp. of dry oregano

- 4 lb. of b2 in pork shoulder

- 3 tbsp. of smoked paprika

- 2 tbsp. of chili powder

- 2 tbsp. of sea salt

- bbq-sauce

Directions:

1. Aside from the BBQ-Sauce and pork shoulder, combine all the Ingredients: in a bowl and mix well to make the spice-rub.

2. Rub the spice-rub all over the pork.

3. Tightly wrap the spice covered pork in a plastic wrap; refrigerate it for a minimum of 3 hours or up to 3 days.

4. Unwrap the meat; put it in the crock pot, add ¼ cup of filtered water; and place crock pot on a low heat and cook the meat for about 8-10 hours till it becomes fork-tender.

5. Transfer the meat to a cutting board. Empty the remaining liquid from the crock pot.

6. Pull the pork apart by tearing it into shreds using 3 forks.

7. Place the shredded pork back into the crock pot and cover it with BBQ Sauce

8. Continue to cook on a low heat for a further 3060 minutes till hot. Then serve and enjoy.

Wheat-Belly Chocolate Chip Cookies

Ingredients:

- Baking soda 1 teaspoon

- Almond meal/flour 4 cups

- Sour cream or coconut milk 1/4 cup

- Vanilla extract 2 teaspoons

- Sea salt 1/2 teaspoon

- Dark chocolate chips 10 ounces

- Eggs 4

- Butter 1/2 cup, melted

- Liquid stevia 1/2 teaspoon

Directions:

1. Set the oven to 350 degrees F.

2. Get a baking tray and line it with parchment paper.
3. Get a large bowl and add the baking soda, sea salt, and almond meal/flour. Mix well.
4. Get a medium bowl and mix in the coconut milk, butter, eggs, stevia, and vanilla extract.
5. Combine the 3 bowls and mix well. Add the chips, and blend the cookie dough well.
6. Get a tablespoon-full of the cookie mix and put it on the baking tray, then form it into a cookie shape.
7. Bake the cookies until their edges are colored brown around 25 minutes. Allow to cool before serving.

Mexican Tortillas

Ingredients:

- 2 Eggs

- Almond meal or flour 4 tablespoons

- Fine sea salt 1/4 teaspoon

- Golden flaxseeds 1 cup, ground

Directions:

1. Set the oven to 350 degrees F.

2. Get a baking tray and line it with parchment paper.

3. Get a medium bowl and add the almond meal or flour, sea salt, and flaxseeds into it. Mix well.

4. Add the eggs into the mixture and whisk well.

5. Divide the dough mixture into four equal parts. Form each into a ball.

6. Between 2 pieces of parchment paper, roll each dough ball until you have 6-inch round tortillas.
7. Put the tortillas on the baking tray.
8. Bake the tortilla until they turn golden brown in color about 5 minutes.

Creamy Chocolate Mousse

Ingredients:

- ½ cup whole milk

- 1/3 cup raw h2y

- 1/3 cup unsweetened cocoa powder

- 3 medium avocadoes, pitted and chopped

- 2 teaspoons vanilla extract

Directions:

1. Place the chopped avocado in a food processor and blend smooth.
2. Add the milk, h2y, cocoa powder and vanilla extract.
3. Blend the mixture until smooth and well combined then spoon into dishes.
4. Chill the mousse until ready to serve.

Cinnamon Baked Bananas

Ingredients:

- ½ teaspoon ground cinnamon

- 2 tablespoons grass-fed butter, chopped

- 4 large bananas, peeled and sliced

- 2 tablespoons fresh lemon juice

- 2 tablespoons raw h2y

Directions:

1. Preheat the oven to 400°F and grease a small glass baking dish.
2. Spread the banana slices in the dish and toss with the lemon juice, h2y, and cinnamon.
3. Dot the butter over the bananas and bake for 10 to 15 minutes until tender.

Mushroom Quiches With Mini Kale

Ingredients:

- 1 cup kale, trimmed and torned

- 2 free roaming eggs

- ½ teaspoon dried rosemary, pulverized

- Flaked ocean salt and black pepper, to taste

- ½ cup parmesan cheese, ground

- 1 teaspoon additional virgin olive oil

- ½ cup mushroom, cut

- ½ tablespoon unsweetened coconut cream or coconut milk

Directions:

1. Preheat the oven to 375° F. Gently, oil a 6 cups biscuit plate. In a pan, warm oil on medium warmth. Include mushrooms and sauté for around 4 to 5 minutes. Move the mushrooms on a plate. In the same pan, include kale and sauté for 3 to 4 minutes or until simply shrivelled.

2. Take from warmth. In a dish, include eggs, rosemary, salt and black pepper and beat well. Include mushrooms, kale, cheese and cream in egg mixture and mix until all around joined. Place the mixture in arranged biscuits plate. Prepare for 20 to 22 minutes or until a toothpick embedded in the middle comes out clean. Serve these quiches with crisp greens.

Mushroom Frittata With Broccoli

Ingredients:

- 8 ounces cremini mushrooms, cut

- 2 cups broccoli florets

- 1 teaspoon ocean salt

- ½ teaspoon ground black pepper

- 1 cup destroyed sharp Cheddar cheese

- 2 cups cream

- 1 clove garlic, daintily cut

- 1 teaspoon additional virgin olive oil

- 6 eggs

- 2 tablespoons approximately pressed new dill, slashed

Directions:

1. Preheat the oven to 375°F. Oil a 9" pie plate. In a little skillet, cook the garlic in the oil over medium-low warmth for 3 minutes. Evacuate the garlic and put aside. Build the warmth to medium. Cook the mushrooms, blending habitually, for 8 minutes, or until brilliant.

2. In the interim, put a steamer wicker bin in an expansive pot with 2" of water over medium-high heat. Steam the broccoli for 3 minutes, or until brilliant green and delicate fresh. Remove what's more and generally slash.

3. Add the broccoli to the skillet. Mix to coat. Sprinkle with salt and pepper. Expel from the warmth, and include the saved garlic. Line the base of the pie plate with the vegetables. Top with the cheese.

4. In a dish, whisk together the cream and eggs. Add the dill and race to join. Deliberately pour over the cheese and vegetables.
5. Place the pie plate on a baking sheet and prepare in the focal point of the oven for 35 minutes, or until a knife embedded in the middle comes out clean.

Basic Wheat Free Bread

Ingredients:

- 1 teaspoon cinnamon optional

- ¼ teaspoon ocean salt

- 5 eggs, differentiated

- ¼ cup butter, liquefied

- 1 tablespoon buttermilk

- 1 tablespoon xylitol or 4 drops fluid stevia or to coveted sweetness

- 1¼ cups whitened almond flour

- ¼ cup + 2 tablespoons garbanzo bean chickpea flour

- ¼ cup ground brilliant flaxseeds

- 1½ teaspoons baking soda

Directions:

1. Preheat the oven to 350°F.

2. Oil a 8½" × 4½" pan. In a sustenance processor, consolidate the almond flour, garbanzo bean flour, flaxseeds, preparing pop, cinnamon if utilizing, and salt.

3. Beat until very much mixed. Include the egg yolks, butter, buttermilk, and Xylitol or stevia and heartbeat just until mixed.

4. In an expansive bowl and utilizing an electric blender on high, beat the egg whites until the delicate tops structure.

5. Fill the flour mixture and heartbeat until the egg whites are equitably dispersed, at the same time, don't run the machine at a steady speed.

6. Spread into the pan and prepare for 40 minutes, or until a wooden pick embedded in the middle comes out clean.

7. Cool in the pan for 10 minutes.

Wheat Free Basic Focaccia

Ingredients:

Flavored oil ingredients:

- 2 large garlic cloves, minced

- 1–2 tablespoons minced fresh herbs such as basil or rosemary

- Add 3 tablespoons of olive oil

- ½ teaspoon fine sea salt

Dough ingredients:

- 2 teaspoons baking powder

- ½ teaspoon fine sea salt

- 1 cup buttermilk

- 1 teaspoon instant rapid rise yeast optional

- 4 egg whites

- 2 cups almond meal/flour

- 1 cup garbanzo bean chickpea flour

- ½ cup ground golden flaxseeds

Directions:

1. In a small saucepan over low heat, combine the oil, salt, and garlic and simmer for 10 minutes.

2. Remove the saucepan from the heat.

3. Apply a delicate herb, such as basil, add it to the oil after you swallow the oil from the groove. If using a hardier herb, such as rosemary, allow it to simmer for the full 10 minutes.

4. Set aside for later use. Alternatively, you can go over this step and brush the focaccia with plain olive oil, then sprinkle your favorite seasonings on top.

5. Preheat the oven to 400°F. Grease a 13" × 9" baking sheet with half of the oil, seam it with

6. Parchment paper, and then generously brush the paper with the reserved oil.

7. In a large bowl, blend the almond meal/flour, garbanzo bean flour, flax seeds, baking powder, and salt. Stir or whisk to blend and split up the flour.

8. In a small bowl or glass measure, whisk the buttermilk and yeast, if using, until the yeast dissolves. Set aside for later use. In a separate bowl, whip the egg whites with mixer until stiff peaks form.

9. Add the yeast mix to the flour mixture and shake until a rough dough ball forms.

10. Gently fold in the egg whites until they're fairly well integrated.

11. The dough will not become totally smooth, and the whites will still be slightly frothy.

12. Spread the dough in the pan with a spatula or spoon. Lightly coat your fingertips with cooking spray or dip them into the reserved oil and dimple the top of the bread. Pour the remaining oil mixture over the upper side of the dough, making certain it is totally covered. Oil will pool in the dimples.

13. Bake for 20 minutes or until golden and slightly spongy in the centre. With a pizza cutter or knife, cut into the desired size and number of flat breads. Serve while still slightly warm.

Toad In A Hole Meat Version

Ingredients:

- 2 sausage patties, actually you have a choice on the kind of patty to use, make some beforehand, if you want thaw it if they're still frozen

- 1 tbsp. butter

- 2 large eggs

- Salt and pepper

Directions:

1. Using a knife, cut a hole in the patty. This is where you're going to have the egg, so choose the diameter as you want.

2. Heat the butter on a non-stick pan and fry the patties until it is brown on both sides. Make sure that it lies flat on the pan.

3. Crack the eggs into the holes on the patties if you wanted a scrambled version, beat the eggs with the salt and pepper before pouring them into the hole. Allow the white to set completely for around 2 minutes.

4. Season with salt and pepper. Quickly flip the patties to heat the other side of the egg-in-patty pieces. After a few seconds, slide into a plate and serve immediately.

Sausage And Ham Roll

Ingredients:

- 16 oz. cheese sauce

- 15 pieces of ham slices

- 12 oz. spicy pork sausage, ground

- 12 oz. pork sausage, ground

Directions:

1. Mix and cook the ground sausages in a large skillet over medium high flame until slightly brown.
2. Drain the sausage and mix in the cheese sauce.
3. Spoon some of the ground sausage mixture into a slice of ham and roll it up, securing it with a toothpick.
4. Fry the rolls until the ham are well-cooked.

5. Arrange on a plate and serve with some dip or poured with sauce.

Paleo Pumpkin Bread

Ingredients:

- ¼ tsp Celtic sea salt

- 1 tbsp ground cinnamon

- ½ tsp cloves

- 2 tbsp honey

- 3 large eggs

- 1 cup blanched almond

- ½ tsp baking soda

- 1 tsp nutmeg

- ½ cup roasted pumpkin

- ¼ tsp stevia

Directions:

1. Combine the spices such as cinnamon, cloves, nutmeg, and cloves along with the almond flour and salt in a food processor.
2. Blend few times then add the stevia, pumpkin, eggs and honey.
3. Transfer the batter into a loaf pan.
4. Bake for 45 minutes at 350 degrees.
5. Allow to cool for an hour before slicing.
6. Serve alone or with your favorite spread.

Chocolate Zucchini Bread

Ingredients:

- ¾ cup grated zucchini

- ¼ cup cacao powder

- ½ tsp baking soda

- 2 tbsp coconut oil

- ¼ tsp vanilla stevia

- 1 ¼ cups blanched almond flour

- ¼ tsp Celtic sea salt

- 2 large eggs

- ¼ cup honey

Directions:

1. Mix the cacao powder and almond flour in a food processor.

2. Blend in the baking soda and salt.

3. Add the eggs, honey, stevia, zucchini and coconut oil. Process few more times.

4. Transfer to a greased pan that is dusted with almond flour.

5. Bake in the oven for 40 minutes at 350 degrees.

6. Allow to cool for 2 hours before serving.

Paleo Banana Bread

Ingredients:

- 3 large eggs

- 1 tbsp honey

- 2 cups blanched almond flour

- 1 tsp baking soda

- 3 mashed bananas

- 1 tbsp vanilla extract

- ¼ cup palm shortening

- ½ tsp Celtic sea salt

Directions:

1. Place the bananas, shortening, honey, vanilla and eggs in a food processor.
2. Blend the Ingredients: together until smooth.

3. Add the salt, almond flour and baking soda then process again.

4. Scoop the batter and place on the greased loaf pan.

5. Remove from the heat and place on top of the counter to cool.

6. Serve with your favorite coffee.

German Apple Pancake

Ingredients:

- 1/4 cup coconut flour

- 1/2 teaspoon baking soda

- 1/8 teaspoon nutmeg

- 2 apples, cored and diced

- 2 tablespoon coconut oil

- 2 tablespoon raw organic honey

- 1 teaspoon cinnamon

- 1 teaspoon nutmeg

- juice of 1/2 lemon

- 6 eggs

- 1 cup almond milk

- 3 tablespoon coconut oil, melted

- 2 teaspoon vanilla

- 2 teaspoon pure maple syrup

- handful of crushed pecans

Directions:

1. Preheat Oven to 425°F.

2. In a large bowl, whisk eggs, almond milk, coconut oil, vanilla, and maple syrup. In a small bowl, stir coconut flour, nutmeg, and baking soda.

3. Mix dry Ingredients: into wet Ingredients: and beat well to combine, set aside while you prepare the apples.

4. In a small frying pan, heat 2 tablespoon coconut oil and raw organic honey. Stir in cinnamon and nutmeg and juice of 1/2 Lemon and cook for 1 minute.

5. Add in your apples and sauté until all your apples are nicely coated.

6. Evenly divide your apple mixture between 8 ramekins greased with coconut oil and then evenly divide your egg mixture on top of the apples between the 8 Ramekins.

7. Place your Ramekins on a baking sheet and bake for 20 minutes at 425 and then reduce heat to 375˚F and cook for an additional 20 minutes. Sprinkle with pecans when removed from the oven.

Chocolate Coffee Coconut Truffle Desserts

Ingredients:

- 1 tablespoon unsweetened coconut flakes

- 1/2 teaspoon raw honey

- 1 tablespoon coconut oil

- 1/2 cup coconut butter

- 3 tablespoons 100% cocoa powder

- 1 tablespoon ground coffee

Directions:

1. Melt the coconut butter in a microwave so that it can be mixed with a fork.
2. Mix in all the Ingredients: except the coconut oil and mix well with a fork.

3. Take an ice-cube tray and pour approximately 1/4 teaspoon of coconut oil into 6-7 of the cups.
4. Spoon the mixture into each cup of the ice-cube tray and gently pat them flat with a fork. Freeze for 4-5 hours.
5. Defrost at room temperature for 15-20 minutes before serving.

All In One Mushroom Curry

Ingredients:

- 1 large potato

- 1 eggplant

- 250g button mushrooms

- 150ml vegetable stock

- 400ml coconut milk

- 1 tablespoon of olive oil

- 1 onion

- Fresh coriander

- Curry paste

Directions:

1. Chop the onion into large pieces. Peel and dice the potato.

2. Peel and dice the eggplant into sizeable chunks.
3. In a saucepan, heat the tablespoon of olive oil for a moment.
4. Fry on a low temperature for roughly 5 minutes or until the potato has begun to soften.
5. Add in the eggplant and button mushrooms and fry for another 2-3 minutes.
6. Combine the vegetable stock, curry paste and coconut milk with the contents of the saucepan.
7. Boil for 10 minutes and mix in the fresh coriander before serving.

Dump Dinner Mushroom & Rice

Ingredients:

- 2 teaspoon of rosemary

- 250g chestnut mushrooms

- 2 red bell peppers

- 400g chopped tomatoes

- 425ml vegetable stock

- 200g basmati rice

- 1 tablespoon of olive oil

- 1 large onion

- Fresh parsley

Directions:

1. Preheat your oven to 380F or gas mark 5.

2. Wash the basmati rice using water from your tap and a sieve.

3. Peel and dice the onion and slice the chestnut mushrooms into quarters.

4. Slice the red bell peppers into thin strips.

5. In a large saucepan, heat the tablespoon of olive oil for a moment then add the chopped onion and fry for 5 minutes.

6. Add the mushrooms and rosemary to the casserole dish, mix then fry for 2-3 minutes.

7. Next add the remaining Ingredients:, except for the parsley and stir thoroughly.

8. Bring the saucepan to the boil, cover and leave to simmer for 25 minutes. Dust with parsley to serve.

Crepes With Ricotta And Strawberries

Ingredients:

Filling

- 1 teaspoon lemon peel

- 2 cups strawberries, halved

- 1 cup ricotta

- 1 teaspoon xylitol or 1 drop liquid stevia or to desired sweetness

Crepes

- ¼ teaspoon sea salt

- 1½ cups almond or carton-variety coconut milk

- 4 eggs

- ¼ cup coconut flour

- ¼ cup golden flaxseed meal

- ¼ teaspoon vanilla extract

Directions:

To prepare the filling:

1. In a small bowl, mix the ricotta, Xylitol or stevia, and lemon peel and then set aside for later use.

To cook the crepes:

2. In a large bowl, mix the coconut flour, flaxseed meal, and salt. In a modest bowl, whisk together the milk, eggs, and vanilla. Now, add the egg mixture to the flour mixture and stir until combined.

3. Coat a small nonstick frying pan with oil and heat over medium high temperature.

4. Measure ⅓ cup of the Batter and pour into the pan, swirling the batter around so it coats the underside of the pan.

5. Cook for 3 minutes, or until the tip of the crepe looks dry.

6. Move around the crepe and cook for 1 min, or until the bottom is dry.

7. Repetition with the remaining batter, stacking the Crepes as they are prepared.

8. Top each crepe with 2 tablespoons of the ricotta filling and ¼ cup of the strawberries.

Beef And Arugula Sandwiches

Ingredients:

- 4 slices Basic Focaccia

- 4 cups baby arugula

- 4 roasted red peppers, patted dry
  and thin into slips

- 12 ounces sliced cooked steak or
  roast beef

- ¼ cup sour cream

- 2 tablespoons extra virgin olive oil

- 1 tablespoon red wine vinegar or
  apple cider vinegar

- 1 tablespoon prepared horseradish

Directions:

1. In a modest bowl, whip together the sour cream, oil, vinegar, and horseradish until blended.
2. On each of 4 lunch plates, place 1 slice of focaccia.
3. Equally divide the arugula, peppers, and steak or roast beef among the focaccia.
4. Drizzle with the horseradish sauce.

Butternut Bisque

Ingredients:

- 2 cloves garlic, minced

- ½ teaspoon ground red pepper

- ½ teaspoon ground cumin

- 2¼ cups chicken juices

- ¼ teaspoon ocean salt

- ¼ teaspoon ground black pepper

- ¼ cup entire plain yogurt or sour cream

- 1 expansive butternut squash

- 2 tablespoons butter or coconut oil + 2 tablespoons butter discretionary

- 2 medium onions, slashed

- 1 medium red bell pepper, slashed

Directions:

1. Pierce the squash a few times with a sharp knife; place it on a paper towel in the microwave oven.
2. Microwave on high power for 5 minutes.
3. Divide the squash longwise also, uproot and dispose of the seeds; microwave on high power for 5 minutes. Put aside to cool somewhat.
4. In a huge pot over medium-high warmth, warm 2 tablespoons of the butter or oil.
5. Cook the onions, bell pepper, and garlic, mixing periodically, for 5 minutes.
6. Scoop the squash tissue from its shell and cut into lumps; include the squash pieces, ground red pepper, cumin, and stock to the soup.
7. Heat to the point of boiling. Lessen the warmth to medium low.

8. In the event that sought, include 2 tablespoons of butter for a wealthier taste.

9. Cover and stew for 15 minutes. Exchange the soup to a blender or nourishment processor.

10. Puree until smooth. Return the soup to the saucepan.

11. Blend in the salt and black pepper. Warmth through. Enhancement every presenting with yogurt or sour cream.

Fennel And Apple Soup

Ingredients:

- 2 huge fennel bulbs, uprooted stems and cut

- 2 cups sans gluten chicken broth

- 2 tablespoons new basil, cleaved

- Flaked ocean salt and black pepper, to taste

- 2 tablespoons additional virgin olive oil

- 1 onion, hacked

- 2 substantial fruits, peeled, cored and cut

Directions:

1. In an extensive soup pan, warmth oil on medium-low warmth. Include onion and sauté for 8 to 10 minutes.

2. Include apple and fennel and cook, blending for around 8 to 10 minutes.

3. Include basil and chicken broth. Cook for 2 minutes and let it cool marginally.

4. In a sustenance processor, include soup and mix in bunches until rich and smooth.

5. Move the soup in pan once more. Heat the soup totally before serving.

6. Top this soup with crisp coriander leaves and avocado slices.

Blueberry Almond Crisp

Ingredients:

- ¼ cup almonds, finely chopped

- ½ teaspoon ground cinnamon

- 6 tablespoons grass-fed butter, chopped

- 6 cups fresh blueberries

- 1 tablespoon coconut flour

- 1 cup almond flour

Directions:

1. Preheat the oven to 375°F and grease a round pie plate.
2. Toss the blueberries with the coconut flour then spread them in the pie plate.
3. Whisk together the almond flour, almonds and cinnamon in a mixing bowl.

4. Cut in the butter until you are left with a crumbly mixture.

5. Spread the crumbly mixture over the blueberries.

6. Bake for 18 to 20 minutes until hot and bubbling.

Lemon Coconut Cupcakes

Ingredients:

- ½ cup raw honey

- ¼ cup fresh lemon juice

- 1 tablespoon fresh lemon zest

- 1 teaspoon vanilla extract

- ½ cup shredded unsweetened coconut

- ¾ cups blanched almond flour

- 2/3 cup sifted coconut flour

- 1 ½ teaspoon baking soda

- ½ teaspoon salt

- ¾ cups unsweetened applesauce

Directions:

1. Preheat the oven to 350°F and line a muffin pan with paper liners.

2. Combine the flours, baking soda and salt in a mixing bowl.

3. In another bowl, whisk together the applesauce, honey, lemon juice, eggs and vanilla extract.

4. Stir the wet Ingredients: into the dry until combined then fold in lemon zest and coconut.

5. Spoon the batter into the muffin pan, filling each cup ¾ full.

6. Bake for 20 to 25 minutes until a knife inserted in the center comes out clean.

7. Cool the cupcakes for 5 minutes in the pan then turn out onto a wire rack.

Strawberry Cream Pie

Ingredients:

Crust:

- Egg 1 large piece

- Almond meal or flour 1½ cups

- Butter 4 ounces, melted

- Cinnamon 1 teaspoon, ground

- Salt ½ teaspoon

Cream filling:

- Sweetener 1/2 cup

- Vanilla extract 1 teaspoon

- Cream cheese 8 ounces, at room temperature

- Sour cream 8 ounces

Gelatin topping:

- Sweetener 1 cup

- Ice 1 cup, crushed

- Gelatin 1 packet, or 2 1/2 teaspoons

- Strawberries 6 ounces, fresh/frozen, chopped

- Water 1½ cups

Directions:

1. Let`s start with the crust. Get a medium bowl and add in the almond meal, salt, and cinnamon. Mix well.

2. In the same bowl, add the egg and butter, and whisk thoroughly. This serves as the dough.

3. Get a pie plate 9 inches and grease it with some oil. Place the dough into the plate and spread it using a large spoon.

4. In an electric mixer, add in all the Ingredients: for the cream filling, and whip for about 3 minutes.
5. Pour the cream filling over the pie crust.
6. Refrigerate in the freezer for about 30 minutes.
7. Get a medium saucepan and add in the water, then the gelatin. Let the mixture sit for 5 minutes.
8. Place the saucepan over low heat, and then add the sweetener. Heat until the gelatin has dissolved. Do not boil.
9. Add in the strawberries.
10. Remove the saucepan from heat. Pour the crushed ice into it.
11. Allow the gelatin topping to cool for about 30 minutes.
12. Over the cream pie, pour the cooled gelatin mixture.

13. Cool the cream pie in the refrigerator for at least 2 hours or overnight. Then serve.

Raisin Crunch Bars With Nuts

Ingredients:

- Coconut 2 cups, unsweetened, and shredded

- Whey protein 1 cup

- Sweetener ½ cup

- Sea salt ¼ teaspoon

- Water ½ cup

- Coconut oil ¼ cup, melted

- Almond butter ½ cup, at room temperature

- Walnut fragments ½ cup

- Raisins ½ cup dried

- Pumpkin seeds ½ cup, raw

- Cinnamon 2 teaspoons, ground

- Vanilla extract 1 teaspoon

Directions:

1. Set the oven to 300 degrees F.
2. Get a baking tray and line it with parchment paper.
3. In a large bowl, mix the coconut and cinnamon well.
4. In a small bowl, add in the coconut oil and vanilla extract and then mix well.
5. Combine the two bowls and mix thoroughly.
6. Put the mixture onto the baking tray and spread it thinly.
7. Bake the mixture for around 5 minutes.
8. Remove from the oven and toss it with a spoon.

9. Put it back to the oven and heat it until it turns light brown in color about 2 to 3 minutes.

10. Place the toasted coconut back into the large bowl, then add the pumpkin seeds, almond butter, raisins, walnuts, whey protein, salt, sweetener, and water. Mix well.

11. Put the mixture onto a parchment paper-surface, then shape it into bars.

12. Store the bars into the refrigerator.

Flourless Choco Cake

Ingredients:

- 2 tablespoons of butter salted

- 2 large sized eggs yolks separated; at room temperature

- 2 oz of bittersweet choco 60%-70% cacao

- 1 to ½ tablespoons of sweetener you can use the wheat free market brand

Directions:

1. Preheat your oven to 350 degrees F.
2. Put the chocolate and butter in your double broiler. Allow the chocolate to melt then once done, turn off the heat and add sweetener. Remove from stove and add in the egg yolks. Keep on whisking. This will make it thick.

3. Using a separate bowl, whip the egg whites until it reached a stiff peak consistency. Fold in the chocolate mixture carefully and don't overwork it.

4. Brush some butter at the side and bottom of the 2 ramekins. Sprinkle about a half a teaspoon of sweetener on each ramekin then pour the batter evenly on both.

5. Bake for about 18-20 minutes or until the middle is already cooked. Serve with whip cream on top if you want. Enjoy!

Brownie Bites

Ingredients:

- 3 tablespoons of sweetener

- 1 large sized egg

- 3 tablespoons of heavy cream you can also use coconut milk

- 3 tablespoons of melted butter unsalted

- 1/8 teaspoon of sea salt

- 1 teaspoon of vanilla extract

- ¼ cup of cacao powder raw; you may also use unsweetened cocoa powder

- 1 cup of baking mix all purporse

- ¼ cup of walnuts or pecans chopped

- Dark choco chips and extra nuts for topping optional

Directions:

1. Preheat your oven to 325 degrees F.
2. Grease your muffin pan using the butter then set it aside.
3. Using a medium sized bowl, combine cocoa powder, baking mix, sweetener and salt. Whisk them well together then add in the cream, butter, vanilla, egg and nuts. Mix until it is combined well.
4. Scoop and divide the batter on the muffin pan. You can add dark choco chips or nuts on top before cooking.
5. Bake for about 9 to 11 minutes. Bring out of the oven and let cook for about 2 minutes. Serve and enjoy!

Bacon-Wrapped Chicken Pops

Ingredients:

- 8 slices uncured bacon

- 1 pc. jalapeno seeds removed, finely chopped

- 4 pcs. chicken fillet tenderized and cut into two

- 1.5 oz. cream cheese

Directions:

1. Lay the chicken fillets flat.
2. Spread a small amount of cream cheese on each fillet and sprinkle with chopped jalapeno pepper..
3. Roll the chicken fillet and then wrap with a piece of bacon. Secure with a tooth pick.
4. Place the chicken pops on the grill and cook until the bacon is brown and crispy.

No-Sweat Baked Salmon

Ingredients:

- 2 slices of organic butter

- ½ lemon cut into thin slices

- 16 oz. Salmon fillet

- Salt and pepper to taste

Directions:

1. Preheat oven at 325°F
2. Lay the salmon on a tin foil big enough to wrap the fillet
3. Top the fish with lemon and slices of butter.
4. Season with salt and pepper.
5. Wrap the salmon on a foil and cook in the oven for 30 minutes.

Baked Chicken Ginger

Ingredients:

- ½tbsp. oyster sauce

- 1½tbsp. light. Soy sauce

- 1 tbsp. raw honey

- 1 tsp. sesame oil.

- 1½ tsp. white pepper

- 16 oz. chicken legs

- 1 2"ginger peeled, finely chopped

- 5 garlic cloves chopped

- salt to taste

Directions:

1. Place the chicken legs in a large bowl and rub
   with ginger and garlic. And then add the rest

of the Ingredients: in the bowl. Mix well. Make sure that the chicken is well-coated with the marinade.

2. Set aside for 30 mins. minimum inside the fridge.

3. Heat oven at 375°F. Place the drumsticks on a lined baking sheet and cook for 35 mins. or until the chicken skin turns golden brown.

Coconut Flapjacks

Ingredients:

- 3 eggs

- ½ cup almond or container assortment coconut milk

- ½ cup water

- 1 teaspoon vanilla

- 2 tablespoons butter, dissolved

- ¼ cup coconut flour

- ¼ cup almond meal

- 1 teaspoon baking soda

- 1 tablespoon xylitol or ¼ teaspoon fluid stevia or to wanted sweetness discretionary

Directions:

1. Preheat a frying pan over medium warmth. In an expansive dish, consolidate the coconut flour, almond dinner, and baking soda. In a little bowl, whisk the eggs.

2. Include the milk, water, vanilla, butter, and xylitol or stevia on the off chance that utilizing, and whisk well.

3. Empty the egg mixture into the flour mixture and blend until consolidated.

4. Oil a skillet or frying pan and warm over medium warmth. For every pancake, pour ¼ cup of batter onto the frying pan.

5. Cook for 2 to 3 minutes, or until the air pockets structure and the edges are cooked.

6. Turn and cook for 2 minutes, or until the underside are daintily seared. Rehash with the remaining batter.

Chopped Chicken Hash

Ingredients:

- 1 medium tomato, hacked

- ½ cup red bell pepper, seeded and slashed

- ½ cup cooked grass-nourished chicken, hacked

- ½ cup spinach, trimmed and torn

- 1 ½ teaspoons additional virgin coconut oil

- 2 cloves garlic, slashed

- 2-3 turnips, peeled and hacked into 3D squares

- ¼ cup onion, cleaved

Directions:

1. Flaked ocean salt and black pepper, to taste

2. In a non-stick pan, warm oil on medium warmth. Include onion and sauté for around 1 moment. Include turnip and cook blending regularly for around 5 minutes.

3. Include onion, tomato and bell pepper and cook, mixing regularly for 5 minutes.

4. Include chicken and cook for 4 to 5 minutes.

5. Include spinach and cook for 2 to 3 minutes or until simply shriveled.

6. Season with salt and black pepper. Serve this hash with poached eggs.

Grilled Salmon Mediterranean Style

Ingredients:

- 1 crushed garlic clove

- 1 tsp. Greek Seasoning or mix and match some of your favorite spices

- 2 salmon pieces, skinless, around 6 oz. each

- 1 ½ tbsp. olive oil

Directions:

1. Mix olive oil, seasoning and garlic in a bowl.
2. Rub the drained salmon pieces with the mixture and let it marinate for around 15 minutes.
3. Heat some olive oil on your grill pan.
4. Then when oil starts to sizzle, cook salmon for 2 to 3 minutes.
5. Rotate the fish a quarter of a turn and cook for another 2 to 3 minutes.

6. Turn over the fish and cook for 1 to 2 minutes more on the other side.

7. The total time that the fish is to cook should not exceed 8 minutes, depending on the heat and the thickness of the salmon pieces.

8. If cooked for more than that, the fish will dry up and turn hard, firm is what you want with cooked fish.

Cod Skillet

Ingredients:

- 2 tbsp. parsley, chopped

- 24 oz. cod, filleted 1 medium-sized zucchini, sliced into quarter-inch cuts

- 1 tbsp. olive oil

- 1 small onion, sliced thinly

- 1 pinch each of salt and freshly ground black pepper

- 3 cloves of garlic, minced

- ½ cup roasted red pepper, sliced thinly

- 14 ½ oz. diced tomatoes, well drained

Directions:

1. Heat oil in a large skillet over medium-high heat.
2. Add onion, garlic, zucchini, salt and pepper. Stirring occasionally, cook for about 10 minutes.
3. Stir in the peppers and tomatoes, letting it simmer on medium heat for 10 minutes more.
4. Lay the fish fillets on the sauce, pouring some on top of the meat and cover.
5. Continue to simmer until the fish is cooked through, around 10 minutes.
6. Sprinkle with freshly chopped parsley and serve warm.

Irish Soda Bread

Ingredients:

- Pinch of caraway seeds

- ¼ tsp Celtic sea salt

- ½ cup raisins

- 2 tbsp apple cider vinegar

- 2 ¾ cup blanched almond flour

- 1 ½ tsp baking soda

- 2 eggs

- 2 tbsp agave nectar

Directions:

1. Mix the baking soda, almond flour, raisins and salt in a bowl.
2. Combine the apple cider vinegar, agave nectar and eggs in a separate bowl.

3. Combine the wet and dry Ingredients:.

4. Place the dough in a parchment paper. Form into a large ball that is approximately 8 inches across and 1 ½ inches tall.

5. Use a knife to scrape half an inch of dough at the top. This should look like a cross.

6. Sprinkle the top with caraway seeds.

7. Place on top of the baking sheet.

8. Bake for 20 minutes at 350 degrees.

9. Turn off the oven but leave the bread inside for 10 more minutes.

10. Allow the bread to cool for 30 minutes before serving.

Sweet Potato Pancakes

Ingredients:

- 2 cups almond flour

- 4 tbsp almond milk

- ½ tsp vanilla extract

- ½ tsp ground cinnamon

- 1 cup mashed sweet potatoes

- 2 eggs

- ½ tsp baking powder

- ½ tsp ground nutmeg

Directions:

1. Combine all of the wet Ingredients: together in a bowl. You can also place it in a food processor and blend it until you have a smooth consistency.

80

2. Combine the dry Ingredients: together. Use a sifter to ensure that they are evenly mixed.

3. Add the dry Ingredients: to the wet and stir.

4. Add coconut oil on the pan.

5. Spoon about 2 tablespoon of batter into the pan and spread it using your fork.

6. Cook for 2 minutes until bubbles appear.

7. Use a spatula and flip the pancakes.

8. Press down the pancake to ensure that the excess batter oozes out of the dough and thickening in a shape of a pancake.

9. Cook the pancake for another minute.

10. Plate it with honey and cinnamon.

Flapjacks

Ingredients:

- ½ cup water

- ½ tsp Celtic sea salt

- ¼ cup agave nectar

- 1 tbsp vanilla extract

- 2 eggs

- ½ tsp baking soda

- 1 ½ cups blanched almond flour

- Grape seed oil for sautéing

Directions:

1. Combine eggs, vanilla, agave and water in a food processor and blend until it is smooth.

2. Add the salt, baking soda and almond flour into the mixture and blend again to incorporate the Ingredients: better.
3. Pour the oil in a pan and place over medium heat.
4. Pour the batter into the pan.
5. Flip the pancake when bubbles start to appear at the surface.
6. Remove from the heat and transfer to a plate.
7. Repeat the process until all of the batter is used.

Blueberry And Blackberry Crumble

Ingredients:

- ¼ cup chopped walnuts

- 4 pitted dried dates

- ½ teaspoon cinnamon

- ¼ teaspoon salt

- ¼ cup coconut oil, melted

- ¼ cup sliced almonds

- 2 cups fresh blueberries

- 2 cups fresh blackberries

- Juice from a fresh lemon

- 1 cup almond flour

Directions:

1. Preheat oven to 350°F.

2. Place the berries in a 9 inch x 9 inch baking dish, and squeeze juice from half of the lemon over and mix.

3. Press the fruit gently into place and rest at room temperature. In a food processor, combine the almond flour, dates, walnuts, cinnamon, and salt.

4. Pulse until combined. Add in the coconut oil and process on high for 5-10 seconds, or until thoroughly combined.

5. Pour topping into a bowl and mix in the sliced almonds.

6. Sprinkle topping over the berries and lightly press into the fruit with a spoon.

7. Bake for 30-40 minutes, until browned.

Fudgy Espresso Brownies

Ingredients:

For the Brownie

- 1 cup Sucanat or palm sugar

- ¼ cup strong hot coffee

- ¼ cup unsweetened cocoa powder

- 2 eggs

- ½ teaspoon baking soda

- ¼ teaspoon salt

- 6 tablespoons non-dairy butter

- 6 ounces chocolate

- 2 tablespoons coconut flour

- ¼ cup plus 2 tablespoons tapioca flour

- Extra butter for pan greasing

For the Mocha Frosting

- ¼ cup strong hot coffee

- ¾ cup Sucanat or palm sugar

- ¼ cup non-dairy butter, melted

- ¼ cup non-dairy butter, softened

Directions:

For the Brownie

1. Preheat the oven to 350°F.
2. Grease an 8x8 baking pan and line with parchment paper.
3. Ensure eggs are at room temperature. You may run them under warm water for about 10 seconds while shelled.
4. Gently melt the semisweet chocolate and butter in a double boiler.
5. You may use the microwave at 50% heat at 30 second intervals with intermittent stirring. Stir

in the coffee and unsweetened cocoa powder. Measure the sugar and coconut flour and add to a food processor. Give a few pulses to make a superfine texture. Sift together the superfine coconut flour, sugar, tapioca flour, baking soda, and salt. Beat the eggs and add the dry Ingredients:.

6. Beat until combined. Add the rest of the wet Ingredients: and beat until incorporated.

7. Pour the batter into the lined 8x8 pan. Bake for 25-30 minutes at 350F until a toothpick inserted into the center of the batter comes out clean. When done, remove from the oven and let cool in the pan for at least 15 minutes.

For the Mocha Frosting

8. Measure the sugar and add to the food processor. Give a few pulses to make a superfine texture. Gently heat the sugar with the ¼ cup of melted butter and coffee until dissolved or mostly dissolved. Refrigerate the

mixture for a few hours. It will look terrible at this stage, but don't despair.

9. It is beneficial, but not necessary, to mix every now and then while cooling.

10. When the mixture is cold enough, beat in the softened butter 1 tablespoons at a time on high speed. I find the hand mixer best for this task.

Dump Dinner Chilli

Ingredients:

- 1 tablespoon of olive oil

- 1 tablespoon chilli powder

- 1 teaspoon cumin

- 1 teaspoon hot sauce

- 1 onion

- 3 sweet potatoes

- 1 jar of salsa

- 450g black beans

Directions:

1. Peel and dice the onion. Dice the sweet potato into sizeable chunks.

2. In a large saucepan, heat the olive oil for a moment over medium heat.

3. Add your sweet potato chunks as well as the chilli powder, cumin and hot sauce.
4. Fry for another 2-3 minutes then add your salsa, vegetable stock and a half a cup of water.
5. Bring the contents of your skillet to the boil and simmer for 5 minutes.
6. Then add your black beans to the saucepan cover and leave to simmer for 20 minutes.
7. Serve warm or store in a container for later.

Chickpea & Potato Curry With Cumin & Turmeric

Ingredients:

- 1 tablespoon of curry powder

- 400g chopped tomatoes

- 2 large potatoes

- 425ml vegetable broth

- 400g chickpeas

- A pinch of salt & pepper

- 1 onion

- 2 garlic cloves

- 1 teaspoon turmeric

- 1 tablespoon of olive oil

- 1 teaspoon ground cumin

Directions:

1. Peel and dice the onion. Peel the potatoes and dice them into sizeable chunks and crush the garlic.

2. In an iron skillet heat the tablespoon of olive oil for a moment.

3. Add in the onion, frying for 5 minutes or until the onions have become golden and soft.

4. Add in the garlic, turmeric, cumin, curry powder as well as a pinch of salt and pepper and fry for 1-2 minutes.

5. Combine the chopped tomatoes, diced potatoes, vegetable broth and chickpeas with the contents of the skillet.

6. Bring to the boil, cover and leave to simmer for 20 minutes.

7. Serve warm or store in a container for later.

Tasty Tomato Soup

Ingredients:

- 2 tablespoons tomato glue

- 1 teaspoon dried basil, pounded

- 1 cup cream or canned coconut milk

- ¼ cup crisp basil, cleaved

- 1 tablespoon additional virgin olive oil

- 1 little onion, cleaved

- 2 cups vegetable or chicken puree

- 1 can 14 ounces diced tomatoes

Directions:

1. In a substantial pan over medium-high warmth, warm the oil.

94

2. Cook the onion, blending at times, for 5 minutes, or until delicate.

3. Include the chicken puree, tomatoes with juice, tomato glue, and dried basil. Heat it to the point of boiling.

4. Diminish the warmth to low, cover, and stew for 20 minutes, or until marginally thickened. Let cool for 10 minutes.

5. Move the mixture in clusters to a blender or nourishment processor.

6. Puree until smooth. Again, put it inside a pan. Include the cream or coconut milk.

7. Cook, mix for 3 minutes, or until warmed and thickened. Decorate with basil and serve hot.

Delicious Shrimp Bisque

Ingredients:

- 1 tablespoon minced crisp parsley

- 2 teaspoons minced crisp dill

- 1 teaspoon lemon juice

- 2 cups chicken or vegetable juices

- 1½ cups creamer or canned coconut milk

- 2 tablespoons butter or additional virgin olive oil

- 1 medium onion, slashed

- ¾ pound peeled and deveined medium shrimp

- 1 cup tomato puree

- Dash of ground red pepper

Directions:

1. In a medium pan over medium warmth, warm the butter or oil.

2. Cook the onion for 5 minutes, or until delicate. Include the shrimp, tomato puree, parsley, dill, lemon juice, and soup.

3. Stew for 10 minutes. Include the cream or coconut milk and the pepper and warmth through. Serve embellished with the chive.

Cauliflower-Cheeseburger Soup

Ingredients:

- 1 tablespoon minced crisp parsley

- ½ teaspoon ocean salt

- ¼ teaspoon paprika

- 1 teaspoon ground black pepper

- 1 tablespoon coconut flour

- ½ cup destroyed sharp Cheddar cheese

- 4 cups chicken broth, isolated

- ½ head cauliflower, cut into florets

- 1 tablespoon butter or coconut oil

- 1 little onion, slashed

- ½ pound ground beef

Directions:

1. In an expansive saucepan, consolidate 3¾ cups of the broth and the cauliflower.

2. Cover and bring to a boil over high warmth. Lessen the warmth to medium-low.

3. Cook for 15 to 20 minutes, or until the cauliflower is delicate when pierced with a fork.

4. Then, in a medium skillet over medium-high warmth, warm the butter or oil.

5. Cook the onion, blending sporadically, for 5 minutes, or until brilliant.

6. Disintegrate in the beef. Cook, blending sporadically, for 8 minutes, or until no more pink.

7. Blend in the parsley, salt, paprika, and pepper. Expel from the warmth and put aside.

8. Exchange the cauliflower mixture to a sustenance processor or blender and puree until smooth.

9. Come back to the saucepan. In a little bowl, whisk the coconut flour with the remaining ¼ cup broth until smooth.

10. Progressively add to the cauliflower mixture and cook, whisking continually, over medium warmth for 3 minutes, or until somewhat thickened.

11. Rush in the cheese just until it dissolves.

12. Expel the pan from the warmth. Mix in the saved beef mixture and serve while hot.

Beef Broth Stew

Ingredients:

- 1 rib celery, daintily cut

- 1 carrot, cut

- 1 teaspoon dried thyme

- ¾ teaspoon ocean salt

- ¼ teaspoon ground black pepper

- 1¾ cups beef broth, partitioned

- 2 pounds peeled butternut squash, cut into 3" pieces

- 2 tablespoons lemon juice

- 2 teaspoons coconut flour

- 2 tablespoons additional virgin olive oil

- 1½ pounds trimmed beef hurl, cut into 1" lumps

- 1 substantial onion, coarsely slashed

Directions:

1. In a Dutch oven over medium warmth, warm the oil.
2. Cook the beef, working in groups if important, for 5 minutes, or until cooked everywhere.
3. Utilizing an opened spoon, exchange the beef to a dish and put aside.
4. Include the onion, celery, and carrot to the pot and cook, blending at times, for 5 minutes, then again until the onion is delicate.
5. Blend in the thyme, salt, and pepper.
6. Return the held beef to the pot. Include 1½ cups of the broth and heat to the point of boiling.
7. Lessen the warmth, cover, and stew for 45 minutes. Blend in the squash and lemon juice.

8. Cover and stew for 30 minutes, or until the meat and squash are delicate.

9. In a little bowl, whisk the coconut flour with the remaining ¼ cup broth.

10. Add to the pot also, cook, mixing continually, for 3 minutes, or until the sauce thickens.

Wheat-Belly Biscuits

Ingredients:

- Cold butter 4 tablespoons, cut into cubes

- Baking powder 4 teaspoons

- Eggs 4, whites only

- Almond flour 1 cup

- Golden flaxseeds 1 cup, ground

Directions:

1. Set the oven to 350 degrees F.
2. Get a baking tray and line it with parchment paper.
3. Get a large bowl. Add the almond flour, baking powder, butter, and golden flaxseeds. Mix well.
4. Get a medium bowl. Pour in the egg whites and beat them on high until soft peaks form.

5. Pour the egg whites into the large bowl mixture. Mix well until it forms a dough.

6. Spoon 8 rounds of the dough onto the baking tray.

7. Flatten each into around ¾-inch circle.

8. Bake the dough pieces until they turn golden brown around 15 minutes. Then enjoy.

Chocolate Almond Biscotti

Ingredients:

- Canned coconut milk OR ricotta cheese 1/2 cup

- Coconut oil 1/4 cup

- Almond milk 1/4 cup, unsweetened

- Almond extract 1 teaspoon

- Almond butter 1/4 cup, at room temperature

- Almonds 1/2 cup, slivered

- Cocoa powder 1/4 cup, unsweetened

- extra-dark chocolate 2 1/2 ounces, chopped

- Eggs 2

- Almond meal/flour 3 cups

- Xylitol 1/4 cup OR any other sweetener

- Coconut flour 2 tablespoons

Directions:

1. Set the oven to 350 degrees F.
2. Get a baking dish and line it with parchment paper.
3. Get a large bowl and pour in the coconut milk, coconut oil, almond milk, almond butter, almond extract, xylitol or sweetener, and the eggs. Whisk thoroughly.
4. Then add the almonds, chocolate, cocoa powder, coconut flour, and almond meal/flour. Stir the mixture well.
5. Pour the mixture into the baking dish and bake for 40 minutes.

6. Remove it from the oven. Reduce the oven`s heat to 300 degrees F, while letting the loaf cool down on a rack for about 15 minutes.

7. Once cool, use a serrated knife to cut the loaf crosswise into ¾-inch slices.

8. Place each slice on its side onto the baking tray.

9. Bake the biscotti slices for 15 minutes. Turn each piece to the other side, and bake for another 15 minutes to make each piece dry and firm.

10. Completely cool the biscotti on the rack for around 30 minutes.

No-Grain Granola Cookies

Ingredients:

- 2 tablespoons of peanut butter

- 2 tablespoons of chocolate chips extra dark

- 2 tablespoons of sweetener

- 2/3 cup of "slow toasted flakes cereal"

- 2/3 cup of classic granola use the wheat free brand

- 2 tablespoons of water

Directions:

1. Preheat your oven to 325 degrees F.

2. Place flakes and the granola on a food processor and pulse until the larger flakes and

nuts are broken down to smaller pieces. Set aside.

3. Using a small sized sauce pan, add water and sweetener.

4. Heat and dissolve the sweetener over low to medium heat.

5. Once dissolved, pour this mixture over the grounded granola and flakes.

6. Add in the chocolate chips and peanut butter. Mix to combine well.

7. Scoop and divide the batter on the muffin pan. Press down the mixture firmly.

8. Bake for about 12 minutes and once done refrigerate for about an hour to set. Serve and enjoy!

Baked Zucchini Sticks

Ingredients:

- 2 tbsp. parsley leaves

- ½tsp. dried oregano

- 2 tbsp. olive oil

- ½cup grated parmesan cheese

- salt and pepper to taste

- 4 pcs zucchini

- ½tsp. dried basil

- ½tsp. dried thyme

- ¼tsp. garlic powder

Directions:

1. Preheat oven at 350˚F.

2. In a bowl, mix the cheese, dried spices, garlic powder, and salt and pepper.

3. Cut the zucchinis into quarters lengthwise and place on a cooling rack coated with a non-stick spray placed on top of a baking sheet.

4. Drizzle the zucchini sticks with olive oil and sprinkle the parmesan and spice mixture.

5. Place in the oven and cook for 15 mins. And then turn the oven into broil and cook for another 2 mins.

Healthy Green Salad

Ingredients:

- ¼ cup cilantro

- 4 strips of uncured bacon Cooked, chopped

- ¼ cup feta cheese

- 2 tbsp. olive oil

- ½tbsp. lemon juice

- 1 bunch romaine lettuce

- 1 pc. avocado pitted, chopped

- 1 small cucumber sliced

- 1 cup cherry tomatoes cut into half

- Salt to taste

Directions:

1. Throw all the vegetables in a bowl and top with bacon and crumbled feta cheese.

2. In a small bowl, whisk the olive oil, lemon juice and salt.

3. Drizzle dressing over the salad. Enjoy!

Pancakes With Lemon-Poppy Seeds

Ingredients:

- 2 teaspoons poppy seeds

- ¼ teaspoon lemon stevia or to fancied sweetness discretionary

- 1½ cups whitened almond flour

- ½ teaspoon baking powder

- ¼ teaspoon baking soda

- ¼ teaspoon ocean salt

- 3 vast eggs, isolated

- 4 tablespoons buttermilk

- 1 tablespoon lemon juice

- 1 tablespoon naturally ground lemon peel

Directions:

1. In a vast dish, whisk together the egg yolks, buttermilk, lemon juice, lemon peel, poppy seeds, and stevia if utilizing.

2. Include the almond flour, baking powder, baking soda, and salt and mix until completely joined.

3. In a little bowl, whisk the egg whites until marginally hardened.

4. Fold into the batter. Oil a skillet or frying pan and warm over medium warmth. For every pancake, scoop 2 piling tablespoons of batter onto the skillet.

5. Cook for 1-2 minutes, or until air pockets structure around the edges.

6. Turn and cook for 1 minute, or until underside is delicately cooked.

7. Uproot to a serving platter. Rehash with the remaining batter, re-lubing the skillet if required.

Coconut-Almond Crunchy Pancakes

Ingredients:

- ¼ cup almond butter, liquefied

- 4 unfenced eggs, beaten

- 1 teaspoon crisp lemon squeeze

- 1 tablespoon normal stevia

- ¼ cup almonds, hacked Extra-virgin coconut oil, for cooking

- ½ cup coconut flour

- ½ cup almond flour

- ½ teaspoon non-aluminium baking soda

- ½ cup almond milk

Directions:

1. In a dish, include flours and baking soda and mix well. In another dish, include butter and milk and beat well.

2. Include eggs, lemon squeeze and Stevia and beat until very much consolidated.

3. Mix egg mixture into flour mixture.

4. Crease in cleaved almonds. In a huge skillet, warm oil on medium warmth. Include a mixture in sought size.

5. Cook for 3 to 4 minutes for each side. Rehash with the remaining mixture.

6. Present with almond or peanut butter.

Greek Souvlaki

Ingredients:

- 1 lb. lamb meat, shoulder part

- 2 tbsp. lemon juice

- ¼ cup olive oil

- 1 tsp. garlic, minced

- 1 tsp. dried oregano, Greek

Directions:

1. Cut the meat into cubes, minimizing the included fat.
2. Combine the rest of the Ingredients: as marinade.
3. Place the meat cubes into the mixture and marinate in the fridge for at least 4 hours, but not too long.
4. Set grill to medium-high heat.

5. Cook meat for 8 to 10 minutes, depending on your preference. Be careful not to over-cook.

Chicken Salad With Peas

Ingredients:

- ¼ cup scallions or green onions, sliced

- 2 cups cooked chicken, diced

- ½ cup frozen green peas or edamame

- ½ cup olives or as much as you prefer

- 3 tbsp. basil

- 1/3 cup mayonnaise

Directions:

1. Thaw the peas and drain in colander.
2. Dice chicken and place them in a bowl, add in the halved olives and the sliced green onions.

3. Paper towel dry the peas and mix in with the others.
4. In a separate bowl, whisk mayonnaise with pesto. Fold into the salad and chill for 1-2 hours before serving.
5. Note: you can also add other Ingredients: to this recipe like bell peppers, radishes, celery, jicama, and cooked asparagus.

Pumpkin Paleo Pancakes

Ingredients:

- ½ cup pumpkin puree

- 2 tbsp honey

- Coconut oil for frying

- 2 tbsp coconut flour

- 2 tbsp vanilla protein powder

- ½ tbsp cinnamon

- ¼ tsp baking soda

- ½ cup almond flour

- 1 tbsp ground flax seed

- Pinch of salt

- 1 tsp pumpkin pie spice

- ¾ cup egg whites

- ½ tsp vanilla extract

Directions:

1. Place the pan over medium heat.

2. Mix all of the dry Ingredients: in a bowl.

3. Whisk the wet Ingredients: together in a bowl.

4. Gently add the wet and dry Ingredients: together.

5. Add enough coconut oil in a pan.

6. Pour the batter and spread it out into a pancake shape.

7. Cook for 4 minutes on the first side and flip. Cook for another 2 minutes.

8. Repeat the process until the batter is used up.

Double Chocolate Cherry Cookies

Ingredients:

- 1 cup dried fruit juice sweetened cherries

- ½ tsp sea salt

- ¼ cup unsweetened cocoa powder

- ¾ cup agave nectar

- 1 cup coarsely chopped dark chocolate

- 1 ½ cups blanched almond flour

- ½ tsp baking soda

- ½ cup grape seed oil

- 1 tbsp vanilla extract

Directions:

1. Preheat the oven. Place parchment papers on the baking sheets.
2. Mix the almond flour, cocoa powder, salt and baking soda in a large bowl.
3. Combine the grape seed oil, vanilla extract and agave nectar in a separate bowl.
4. Combine the wet mixture to the almond flour mixture.
5. Add the cherries and chocolate.
6. Spoon one tablespoon of dough into the baking sheet.
7. Space each cookie about 2 inches from each other.
8. Bake for 15 minutes until the top of the cookies are dry but not overly cooked.
9. Allow the cookies to cool on the rack for 20 minutes before serving.

Chocolate Mug Cake

Ingredients:

- 1 tablespoon unsweetened vanilla almond milk

- ½ tablespoon honey

- 1 egg

- 1 teaspoon vanilla extract

- 1 heaping tablespoon almond flour

- 1 heaping tablespoon unsweetened cocoa powder

Directions:

1. In a mug, mix together all the Ingredients:. Microwave for 1 to 1.5 minutes.

Chili & Pepper Quinoa

Ingredients:

- 1 teaspoon chilli powder

- 1 teaspoon cumin

- A pinch of salt and pepper

- 140g diced green chillies

- 400g chopped tomatoes

- 300ml vegetable broth

- 1 tablespoon of olive oil

- 1 sweet onion

- 2 garlic cloves

- ¾ cup quinoa

- 400g black beans

Directions:

1. Peel and dice the sweet onion. Crush the garlic cloves.

2. In a large iron skillet, heat the tablespoon of olive oil for a moment.

3. Next, add the sweet onion, fry for 5 minutes or until the onion is golden and soft.

4. Add in the crush garlic and fry for another 1-2 minutes.

5. Combine all the remaining Ingredients: into the skillet; bring to a boil, cover and leave to simmer for 20 minutes.

6. Leave to cool for 5 minutes, and then serve.

African Stew

Ingredients:

- 400g chickpeas

- 170g millet

- 1 tablespoon soy sauce

- 115g peanut butter

- 85g kale

- A dash of lemon juice

- 1 tablespoon of olive oil

- 1.4l vegetable stock

- 3 garlic cloves

- 2 onions

- 450g sweet potato

Directions:

1. Peel and dice the onions. Peel and dice the sweet potato.

2. Crush the garlic cloves. Chop the Kale into moderate pieces.

3. Heat the tablespoon of olive oil in a large saucepan for a moment.

4. Next, add the diced onions and fry for 5 minutes or until soft and golden. Add the crushed garlic and fry for a further 1-2 minutes.

5. Add the vegetable stock, sweet potato, millet and soy sauce to the saucepan.

6. Bring to the boil and simmer for 20 minutes.

7. Take 2 tablespoons of the broth and combine with peanut butter.

8. Add this into the saucepan and stir.

9. Finally add the kale and simmer for 3-5 minutes. Serve hot.

Chicken And Wild Rice Soup

Ingredients:

- 2 medium carrots, slashed

- 1 little onion, slashed

- 2 teaspoons lemon-pepper flavoring

- ½ teaspoon ocean salt

- 2 stalks broccoli, cut into little florets 2 cups

- 2 cups creamer

- 6 cups chicken puree

- ½ cup wild rice

- 1 pound boneless, skinless chicken breasts, cubed

Directions:

1. In a vast pot over medium-high warmth, consolidate the chicken puree and rice.

2. Cover and convey to a boil. Decrease the warmth to medium-low and cook for 20 minutes. Include the chicken, carrots, onion, lemon-pepper flavoring, and salt. Cook for 15 minutes.

3. Include the broccoli and cook for 5 minutes, or until the broccoli and rice is delicate.

4. Continuously mix in the creamer.

5. Cook, mixing, for 5 minutes, or until delicate. Serve while hot.

Chicken And Dumplings

Ingredients:

- 2 carrots, cut 2 ribs

- celery, cut

- 3 cups chicken puree

- 1 teaspoon dried thyme

- 1 pack Basic Biscuits wheat free

- ½ container harsh cream or canned coconut milk

- 2 tablespoons spread or coconut oil, isolated

- 8 boneless, skinless chicken thighs

- 2 onions, cleaved

Directions:

1. Preheat the oven to 350°F.

2. In a Dutch oven over medium-high warmth, warm 1 tablespoon of the margarine or oil.

3. Cook the chicken, turning sometimes, for 5 minutes, or until brilliant on all sides.

4. Evacuate to a plate and put aside.

5. Heat the remaining 1 tablespoon spread or oil. Cook the onions, carrots, and celery, blending sometimes, for 5 minutes, or until the onions begin to relax.

6. Include the chicken puree, thyme, the remaining ⅛ teaspoon salt, and the held chicken.

7. Expand the warmth to high. Heat to the point of boiling. Heat, uncovered, for 20 minutes.

8. Meanwhile, prepare biscuits. Take out the Dutch oven from the oven and stir in the sour cream or coconut milk.

9. Increase the oven temperature to 400°F.

10. Dollop 8 biscuits into the chicken mixture. Bake for 15 minutes, uncovered.
11. Cover and bake for 15 minutes, or until a thermometer inserted in the deepest part of the chicken registers 170°F.

Stew Medley With Zucchini

Ingredients:

- ¼ teaspoon crisply ground pepper

- ½ teaspoon oregano

- 4 tablespoons additional virgin coconut oil

- 1 clove garlic, minced

- 1 green bell pepper, daintily cut into julienne strips

- 1 ½ teaspoon chipped ocean salt

- 1 cup meagrely cut onions

- 2 pounds 906 grams zucchini, cleaned daintily and not pared then cut paper thin

- 1 cup diced crisp tomatoes

137

Directions:

1. Heat the oil in a skillet or griddle.

2. Sauté onions and garlic on medium fire for around 5 minutes. Include zucchini and green pepper.

3. Sauté for 10 minutes while blending consistently.

4. Mix in tomatoes, salt, ground pepper, oregano.

5. Cover and cook over low warmth, 20 to 30 minutes while blending at intervals. Serve with your focaccia or basic bread.

Beef Pot Roast With Vegetables

Ingredients:

- 1 can 15½ ounces beef broth

- ½ cup red wine optional

- 1 teaspoon without gluten soy sauce

- 2 teaspoons additional virgin olive oil

- 1 bay leaf

- ¾ pound white turnips, peeled and cut into eighths

- 2 cups solidified pearl onions, defrosted

- 2 cups child carrots

- 2 tablespoons coconut flour

- ¼ cup water

- 1½ pounds boneless beef hurl cook

- ¾ teaspoon dried oregano

- ½ teaspoon dried thyme

- ½ teaspoon ocean salt

- ¼ teaspoon ground black pepper

Directions:

1. Preheat the oven to 400° F.

2. On a work surface, season the beef with the oregano, thyme, salt, and pepper.

3. In a dish, consolidate the broth, wine, and soy sauce. Put aside.

4. In an oven proof pot or Dutch oven over medium-high warmth, warm the oil.

5. Cook the beef for 2 minutes for each side, or until seared.

6. Expel from the warmth and blend in the held broth mixture and inlet leaf.

7.   Cover and prepare for 1½ hours. Include the turnips, onions, and carrots.

8.   Cover and come back to the oven. Prepare for 45 to 55 minutes or until the meat and vegetables are delicate.

9.   With an opened spoon, exchange the beef and vegetables to a serving platter.

10. Set the pot over medium-high warmth. In a little bowl, whisk the coconut flour and water.

11. Step by step add to the pan sauce and cook, whisking always, for 4 minutes, or until thickened.

12. Evacuate the bay leaf and pour the sauce over the beef and vegetables.

www.ingramcontent.com/pod-product-compliance
Lightning Source LLC
Chambersburg PA
CBHW071003120626
46546CB00003B/909